Table of Contents

Advancements in Research and Treatment of Alzheimer's Disease

7. Conclusion

New Treatments for Alzheimer's Disease: An Expert's Perspective

1. Introduction to Alzheimer's Disease

Although it has long been assumed that accumulation of A-beta amyloids in the brain is the primary reason for this disease, in recent years, scientists are increasingly turning their interest to tau protein aggregates as a potentially better candidate for the detection of individuals at risk of developing Alzheimer's. Both of these are discussed in the next chapter, offering a variety of targeted strategies that are currently being scrutinized for their utility as potential solutions. A critical concern is the proper identification of patients with early-stage Alzheimer's disease, including molecular imaging strategies, feasible solutions, and robust biomarkers that are being developed for the diagnosis of sooner, more accurate detection. More broadly, the field is poised to shift paradigms around common conditions of old age where neurological damage is a significant determinant of cognitive difficulties in aging.

Alzheimer's disease is a progressive neurodegenerative disorder that occurs gradually, worsening over time, erasing memory, and preventing a person from handling simple activities of daily living. Alzheimer's may be the ailment that is most probable to lead to the loss of all brain tissues and the most common cause of dementia. However, there is no cure for this illness at this time. Existing medications are merely able to temporarily alleviate the signs and symptoms. Despite over a century of study on Alzheimer's disease, much remains unknown about this affliction, although significant scientific advancements are being accomplished, especially with regard to the medications.

1.1. Overview of Alzheimer's Disease

Alzheimer's disease is the most common and primary cause of dementia worldwide, affecting between 30 to 50 million people today. There are no consistently effective disease-modifying treatments for Alzheimer's disease at this time. It has become increasingly clear in recent years that rather than being entirely genetically-driven (i.e., genetically-determined) as once thought, Alzheimer's disease, like many other neurodegenerative diseases, is multifactorial and driven by a complex mix of genetic, environmental, metabolic, and other (inflammatory, physiological, etc.) factors that can change over one's lifespan as well as across generations.

Alzheimer's disease, also known as AD, is a progressive neurodegenerative disorder first defined by Dr. Alois Alzheimer in the very early 20th century. Alzheimer's disease is associated with the death of numerous nerve cells in many brain regions, often with the region-specific presence of abnormal structures and protein aggregates that can be observed under the microscope. The disease also often contributes to brain shrinkage and a variety of brain-wide biochemical and functional abnormalities that cannot (yet) be traced back to changes in any one individual cell type or network. These changes are thought to account for the wide range of cognitive, personality, and physiological systems that can be impacted in AD patients, including forgetfulness and changes in language, spatial reasoning, planning abilities, personality, and circadian rhythms.

Alzheimer's Disease Introduction

2. Current Challenges in Alzheimer's Treatment

By the time amyloid is detected in the brain, years of underlying pathophysiology have already demonstrated; would we waste time and money on a drug that may temporarily slow things down when a person is already cognitively compromised? The way I see it, there are different ways to prevent Alzheimer's disease. The first pathway is to inhibit the production of amyloid beta peptides in the brain, which eventually form senile plaques. The second pathway is to prevent the tau protein from becoming hyperphosphorylated and forming neurofibrillary tangles. The third pathway is to prevent inflammation. These are strategies currently being used in the drugs being developed.

My belief is that current drugs need to be improved and first-in-class disease-modifying strategies are most likely to work. Let me elaborate. The current drugs for Alzheimer's are not effective; some studies even suggest that we would be better off with nothing at all. This is because the effect of these drugs is minuscule when compared to their high costs. Additionally, when you discontinue these drugs, your cognitive decline returns to the same trajectory, indicating that they are not addressing the underlying pathology of the disease. These same clinical results are observed with the anti-amyloid antibody treatments currently under investigation with the exception being that they are typically given for only a short period of time (i.e., 18 months or so). At best, these drugs slow cognitive decline down but do not stop or reverse it. Clinical trials with BACE inhibitors show that too much is probably too toxic in the brain and they do not work effectively to reduce amyloid. The key, as evident with many other diseases, like cancer for example, is to treat these symptoms early. If we did this, we could potentially limit the damage already done and slow the progression of the disease.

2.1. Limitations of Existing Therapies

This section takes a deeper exploration of the constraints of drugs that are currently licensed to treat Alzheimer's disease.

A major priority in the crisis of dementia is the need for effective symptomatic treatments. At present, only four drugs are licensed in the UK for treating the symptoms of Alzheimer's disease, all of which are categorized as anti-dementia drugs and have diametrically opposed beliefs on the patient care advantages of their use. These drugs, which can, to limited degrees, ameliorate or stabilize the symptoms of Alzheimer's disease, elicit a great deal of hope among families and professionals, all looking to maintain cognitive function and independence for as long as possible. In view of the nature of the disease and the irrefutable levels of global research, it is expected that sure and safe new enhanced medications will be available sooner rather than later, but what are the objections to relying on the currently prescribed drugs and why is us having new treatments such a pressing need? Given the right circumstances, each of these licensed drugs may be useful in our treatment approach, but, similar to many available medications, they are not a panacea and their effects are not uniform.

3. Emerging Therapeutic Approaches

Moreover, strategies that currently are considered as "treatment" need to be reevaluated in wider term. For example, there are now known strategies to block $A\beta$ aggregation, perhaps leading to dimer and/or oligomer dissociation, which could convey a mechanism of action of dimer/oligomer-targeting compounds. Similarly, from the viewpoint of the catecholaminergic hypothesis of AD, the use of L-DOPA was initially part of the "treatment" strategy, however the future use of EGCG, a blocker of the $A\text{-}\beta$ oligomer toxicity, could also be considered as a "treatment." Summarizing these new cognitions indicates an increase of newcoming "treatment" strategies, e.g., against $A\beta$ oligomers, especially dimers.

The field is replete with ongoing and recent efforts from the biotech industry and academia to either modify the underlying disease processes or find new means of alleviating the symptoms of AD. One major line of research is focusing on different targets, as Lu AE58054 does, aside from the cholinergic system that is the main target of present AD drug treatment. For example, two approaches being taken are trying to improve the glutamatergic function with the amyloid in vivo antibody Bapineuzumab and to block the noradrenergic alpha 2 receptor with an amyloid-antibody conjugate. Furthermore, other targets with different rationale are also being tested: Besides both copper and zinc, other metals, which combine with amyloid upshift the Aβ/tau toxicity (in a synergic or in a multiplicative way), more than which could be expected.

3.1. Immunotherapy

Dr. Nicole Maphis, an assistant professor at the University of Kentucky Sanders-Brown Center on Aging, conducts research aimed at harnessing the immune system to target Alzheimer's and tau aggregation. According to Maphis, the advantage of targeting the immune system in therapeutic approaches is the potential protection from the off-target effects of small molecule inhibitors in the brain. The process of phagocytosis and cell clearance is quite complex, so companies generally focus on manufacturing antibodies to target the externalized proteins associated with disease. Helper T-cells may also be used to destroy captured antigen-antibody complexes once they are engulfed, according to Maphis. Immunotherapy primarily targets extracellular proteins related to aberrant mutant gene products, as less is known about antigen presentation of intracellular wild-type proteins.

Immunotherapy aims at treating a disease by adapting or using the immune system. For years, one of the goals in cancer therapy was to do exactly this: harness the body's natural defenses to attack malignant cells. 2011 marked the approval by the Food and Drug Administration (FDA) of the first cancer immunotherapy drug, and the field has received increasing attention and resources for the ensuing decade. Recently, the idea that amyloid plaques could be eliminated with the aid of the immune system has shifted from a radical and speculative idea to a leading candidate in the latest discussions of potential therapeutic targets in Alzheimer's disease. Aducanumab and other proposed amyloid-removing monoclonal IgG antibodies effectively recruit microglia to phagocytose plaques. While some therapies focus on clearing β-amyloid, others address proteins like tau, α-synuclein, or huntingtin aggregates. Paul Aisen, the director of the Alzheimer's Therapeutic Research Institute, takes seriously the idea that the immune system could be a part of combination therapies that are effective for a wider range of neurodegenerative diseases. The degree to which this is the case is still debated.

3.2. Gene Therapy

Drug development in AD has yet to bring to market an agent that has been shown to prevent, slow, or reverse any of the many aspects of the disease. As a result, investment and resources have been concentrated in improving our understanding of the molecular and cellular factors responsible for each of the neuropathological hallmarks of the disease and in finding ways to ameliorate their effects. Here, I will present some promising new routes towards treating Alzheimer's disease through genetic techniques. It has revolutionized the way in which we can address inherited diseases, and neurological and neurodegenerative diseases are major targets. Gene therapy has become increasingly feasible, and the approach is highly specific. It provides a potentially timely intervention, particularly in the context of a disease in which a small genetic change causes a considerable defect. To bring an agent successfully in gene therapy to market, it is essential to have a good pathomechanism. Following that, a good target to manipulate, one that is feasible and can be quantified, is required in a population sufficiently early in the disease course.

Alzheimer's disease (AD) is one of the most common causes of dementia among older individuals living in the developed world. The disease is associated with the accumulation of two proteins within the brain, amyloid and tau. Current treatment strategies focus on relieving symptoms, and a cure is not available. These approaches do not tackle the primary disease-causing mechanisms. To truly address Alzheimer's disease and slow or stop its progression, therapies are being developed to target the underlying disease, both amyloid and tau pathologies in the brain.

4. Clinical Trials and Research Findings

Researchers at the Alzheimer's Research Program at Mayo Clinic, Jacksonville, are using the clinical and pathological diagnostic research criteria to better understand these stages. The ultimate goal of these studies is to reduce or eliminate amyloid and tau from the brains in this stage to prevent or delay cognitive symptoms. The latest findings show that genes that contribute to aging are turned off by switching to the L-VDF metabolic state. In a new clinical trial, participants have undergone 3 separate brain PET scans: one before receiving the vaccine, one just before they receive the annual flu shot, and 1 week before receiving the flu vaccine. The annual flu vaccine causes inflammation in the brain in people with mild Alzheimer's disease. More extensive research looks at glucose metabolism in people with different risk factors for Alzheimer's disease for living well alone and also its impact on predicting cognitive change.

There are many clinical trials being conducted to understand if new drugs or treatments are effective for Alzheimer's disease (AD). The Biogen aducanumab results will be reviewed on March 11, 2021. The combination of low-dose leucine, vitamin D, and omega-3 fatty acids (L-VDF) changes gene expression patterns and improves cognitive and memory function. Genetic testing is being done so we can determine who will benefit from taking L-VDF. Omega-3s will also be tested in people who have already been diagnosed with mild cognitive impairment.

Low-dose lithium and ibuprofen are associated with a decreased risk of Alzheimer's disease. They impact pathways to aging and inhibit inflammation. Higher brain glucose levels are associated with progression from mild cognitive impairment to individuals who develop Alzheimer's disease.

4.1. Key Findings from Recent Studies

Dr. Sano indicated that the development of amyloid imaging has played a major role in uncovering several research developments. A global amyloid scan has also shown that deposits begin earlier than originally thought. Additionally, she emphasized that physical activity is a potential method for reducing disease risk. Dr. Sano highlighted some of the key outcomes from leading studies. These included the 2 monoclonal antibodies donanemab and lecanemab joined their COMPEL and ENGAGE studies, respectively. Aducanumab has been proposed as a new drug that has undergone regulatory confirmation. Predicate reports were published by 2 major pharmaceutical companies, Eli Lilly and Biogen, that studied dose-dependent adverse events. These were both major studies that were negative. No cognitive capacity for donanemab was mentioned by Dr. Sano. In the lecanemab studies, following a 10 mg/kg dosage, a 22% advantage was seen at 78 weeks in one of two identical experiments.

Mary Sano, PhD, director of Alzheimer's Disease Research at the Icahn School of Medicine at Mount Sinai, joined us over 2 days to discuss the highlights of recent research studies and clinical trials. The cause of Alzheimer's disease (AD) is still not well understood, said Dr. Sano. Population risk factors include untreated diabetes mellitus, increasing age, a bad diet, high insulin, head trauma, and a low education level; there is no protection against these factors. As of June 5, 2021, 178 drugs were in clinical trials to improve cognitive function. Patients in the initial phases of cognition, mood, and behavior treatment will not see big improvements in areas where symptoms have never manifested. As dementia progresses, not every area is treated, and the speed of change differs.

5. Potential Future Directions in Alzheimer's Treatment

Alzheimer's disease (AD) is multifactorial. For this reason, there may be a need for several 'antidementia' medications to treat the disease. Additionally, the fact that people can have AD pathologies (e.g. amyloid-β and tau aggregates) without having the symptoms of dementia has led to the hypothesis that some people are resilient to the disease. Treating or preventing AD may require enhancing resilience, possibly in combination with reducing AD pathologies. New ways to identify which antidementia drugs or drug combinations a person may benefit from using, i.e. 'precision medicine', are critical for success. Identification should be based on defining the stage and type of AD pathology and the clinical stage of the disease. Comprehensive assessment including genetic and imaging approaches, molecular biomarkers, and patient history and pathology could be used to this end. Several approaches to preventing and treating AD will be discussed below. The approaches do not include 'alpha-synucleinopathy', which has been shown to coexist with AD in many older adults. It is likely that multimodal approaches, perhaps even use of currently prescribed medications, will be needed to prevent and treat multiple types of dementia.

Although the field of Alzheimer's disease treatment faces challenges and uncertainties, several opportunities exist to identify treatments for this disease in the near future. Prevention of Alzheimer's, including identification of risk factors, will be discussed in the next section. In this section, we focus on treatment. Combining research and clinical experience, we present a series of paths that could lead to future therapeutic discoveries. We begin with the concept of precision medicine—that is, determining the best treatment for a specific patient. We also consider the logical decision-making of each approach as well as the chance that a trial is successful.

5.1. Precision Medicine Approaches

By doing this and further targeting the early inflammatory events and cognitopathological spread of this immune response with replenishing natural inhibitory signaling, we anticipate that this could be one prospective therapy on the horizon in the medium term.

The implication is that the medication(s) would be personalized, not just saying, "There's evidence of inflammation among many risk factors," but instead "Ah, there's evidence of activated microglial inflammation in the right frontal lobe on a T1-weighted PET scan on the FDG." If an individual does not respond to a specific medication but worsens, then we would look at a number of probable "off-target" pathologies still at play or a different/dual pathology not being targeted. This could give opportunities for additional therapeutic options.

The concept of precision medicine essentially posits that healthcare will evolve from a one-size-fits-all approach to a highly individualized or personalized one. In terms of precision medicine for AD, the idea is to screen individuals using biofluids, blood assays, urine markers and neuroimaging and other technologies possibly including functional MRI, PET imaging, perfusion MRI, etc., to gauge what could or should be the best way to treat that person. Treatment would then be given or escalated in those with evidence of inflammation, infection, anaplastic progressing in frontotemporal lobe disease, blunt head trauma idiopathic normal pressure hydrocephalus, vascular contributing to cognitive impairment, encephalopathy, penetrating TBI, obesity, etc.

6. Conclusion and Implications for Patients

The effect of anti-Aβ treatments hinges in part on the extent to which ongoing exposure to additional factors may speed or slow underlying disease progression. Such knowledge should be pursued vigorously, with development of agents that target tau tangles, synaptic loss and neurodegeneration generally. When an arsenal of safe and effective agents with diverse disease-related targets are available for physicians, there will no longer be any benefit in allowing non-amyloid Alzheimer's to run its likely shorter course. Neither patients at risk of PDD, FTLD, or other non-AD neurodegenerations today, nor those several generations into the future, are likely to pose a major ethical problem to this approach. More than anything, seeking out this complexity and facing it may eventually bring the research field into greater harmony with the realities patients face.

In this article, experts in medicine and law discussed several aspects of amyloid-targeted therapy as part of the wider stage investigation in preclinical Alzheimer's disease. Reviewing the comments, certain conclusions and implications for current and future patients can be drawn. First, there is a consensus that addressing amyloid pathology remains an important goal going forward, particularly as we explore the timing and combinations of amyloid-lowering treatments. This goal is based on the large body of evidence that prevails and is supported by the potential benefits for both research and individuals participating in these studies. For both participants in prevention trials and research outcomes, areas of uncertainty and potential risks focus on the potential effects of investigational therapies on cognitive symptoms and not on the need for a more specific diagnostic label.

6.1. Key Takeaways

• Likewise, we conducted two large, multi-center, international trials of ketamine for depression in elderly adults either with or without mild cognitive impairment (MCI) or early Alzheimer's disease (KIDE and ORCHID, respectively). In ORCHID, we did not find efficacy for ketamine, but we did find a very strong behavior-to-treatment effect interaction of ketamine with the quality of the empathic connection between the patient and the research-rater conducting the study. This finding had not emerged in KIDE, possibly because most of the neuroprotective effects of ketamine that it reflected did not last into the future. We are now exploring the replicability and potential pharmacological and other aspects of cutaneous and peripheral vasoconstriction in MCI and AD in a preliminary experiment comparing a combination versus monotherapy of an NMDA receptor antagonist and a sigma1 agonist (in this case, memantine and nerinitian, respectively). This new study, which evolved from our clinical trials, continues our approach of fostering multiple "shots on goal" in treating a complex disorder like Alzheimer's disease.

• We also offer opinions about the various treatment modalities in which we have conducted clinical trials, based on both the results of these experiments and the overall body of work in each field. For instance, in our trial of allopregnanolone, we had a negative trial in women with familial Alzheimer's variants. However, we also found that a blood biomarker seemed to identify people who would actually worsen with the drug, as revealed through a tantalizing signal of improvement in women not affected by the variants. These additional results suggest directions that research on neurosteroids and their modulation could fruitfully take.

• Lack of positive results in clinical trials has led to pessimism about finding treatments for Alzheimer's disease, which can interfere with the implementation of new studies that could lead to promising drug candidates or provide insights into the most likely pathophysiological mechanisms to pursue. In this piece, we briefly recap why we think "there is still hope," including tantalizing findings about connections to other disorders, peculiar dose-related pharmacodynamics of some prior drugs, and better preclinical experiments that lead to more promising clinical trials.

Advancements in Research and Treatment of Alzheimer's Disease

1. Introduction to Alzheimer's Disease

Approximately 5 million Americans, or about 1 in 10 individuals who are at least age 65, have Alzheimer's disease. It has also been estimated that 2 out of 3 people who fall in this age range with Alzheimer's disease are women. The aging of the population is projected to increase the prevalence of Alzheimer's disease to at least 13.8 million older Americans by 2050. The development of treatment and cost-effective treatment modalities for Alzheimer's disease are important because, if the inability to perform daily activities associated with dementia can be delayed even by a small amount, there could be an overall beneficial impact on physical and psychological well-being. Given the major impact Alzheimer's disease has on not only those actually diagnosed with the disease but also their caregivers, treatment for mild cognitive disorder becomes more important. In sum, due to a large, aging population and projected increase in the prevalence of this condition, research into and treatment of Alzheimer's disease is of paramount importance.

Alzheimer's disease is characterized by progressive memory loss and an inability to form new memories. Language problems, disorientation, mood swings, and behavioral issues are some of the common symptoms. The underlying changes in the brain are believed to begin years prior to the manifestation of the first symptoms, resulting in a progressive, permanent neurological condition that results in an inability to perform daily activities.

Alzheimer's disease can have a major impact on not only affected individuals but also their family members and caregivers. It is the sixth leading cause of death in this country. The primary risk factor for developing Alzheimer's disease is increasing age.

1.1. Definition and Symptoms

Certainly, the current research on the disease gives hope to patients and caregivers. In fact, the elucidation of AD pathology combined with the identification of some risk factors, such as age, gender, genetics, reduced physical activity, and obesity, makes it possible to choose new therapeutic targets. Although no disease-modifying drug is available today, several anti-AD medications are currently prescribed but aim to improve some symptoms of the disease for a certain period of time. In the absence of a cure, animal models helping to understand the pathophysiology of the disease and to test new drugs remain essential. Today, the whole world is actively involved in the development of new drugs with nearly 200 new pathways currently being studied. In this book, nine contributions as original articles, systematic reviews, meta-analyses, and reviews, putting AD into the spot of both research and clinical practice, are presented.

Alzheimer's disease is the most common cause of dementia, accounting for 60-80% of dementia cases. It is a progressive neurological disorder that causes a gradual decline in memory and learning, the ability to perform everyday activities, and judgment and decision-making skills. Clinically, signs and symptoms of Alzheimer's disease (AD) progress slowly and in more than 95% of the diagnosed cases, the disease is classified as sporadic or late-onset, with the first signs appearing at 65 years or later. On the other hand, in fewer than 5% of the diagnosed cases, the disease is classified as familial-early onset due to the first signs appearing in their 30s or 40s. Pathologically, AD is characterized by the accumulation of amyloid deposits within the brain in the form of plaques composed of Aβ, neuritic plaques with dystrophic and damaged neuritis, neuropil threads, and neuronal loss. In addition to the Aβ plaques, AD is characterized by hyperphosphorylated tau-containing intracellular deposits in the form of neurofibrillary tangles, neuropil threads, and neuritic profiles. More recently, it has been demonstrated that AD is a multifactorial disease with Aβ and tau pathologies, and that additional contributors are vasculature, lipid transport molecules, autophagy, endosomal and lysosomal function, and the innate and adaptive immune response. AD is associated with a considerable socioeconomic burden due to its increasing prevalence caused by extension of the lifespan and the lack of a cure.

1.2. Prevalence and Impact

Alzheimer's Disease (AD) and related disorders are now one of the leading causes of morbidity and mortality in the western world. Recent data from the Scottish Health Survey 2019 showed that dementia, at 18% of all causes of death, ranks second only to ischemic heart disease (25%). Caught between living longer and complexity of increasing late-life disorders, dementia is now one of the leading causes of disability and dependency among older people worldwide. Clinicians are faced with patients approaching 90 years of age with between four and seven co-morbid diseases, straining public healthcare services and social care. Across the world, the impact of the dementia on the family or carer is significant emotionally, functionally and socio-economically as direct carer costs are higher for AD than cardiovascular and oncologic diseases.

As of 2015, nearly 47 million people were living with dementia globally. As the prevalence of dementia is expected to double every 20 years, it is estimated that the number could rise to 75 million by 2030 and 131.5 million by 2050. For example, Alzheimer's Disease International (ADI) highlighted that one new case of dementia is detected every four seconds. Despite this growing recognition, the extent and impact of dementia on the individual and society is not understood. There is also a widespread misunderstanding of the vast array of symptoms, which include not only cognitive dysfunction and memory loss but also mood and behavior changes. For the general public, dementia signifies an old age pensioner in a nursing home, incapable of independent living, but the recognition of the growing incidents of 'young onset' dementia caused by AD is equally concerning. More research is needed.

2. Understanding the Underlying Causes of Alzheimer's Disease

During the illness progression, many changes in the brain begin to occur because of such a minimal percentage of cases. These changes are frequently characterized by plaques and tangles, which are the accumulation of harmful proteins that have not only been linked to the development of brain cells and communication but also to the presence of Alzheimer's dementia on clinical examinations. The part of the brain responsible for remembering fresh memories is the first to be influenced by these modifications. Each of the plaques and tangles gradually spreads to different places where they may cause harm to the brain and eventually bring harm to some of the already harmed.

When it comes to the underlying causes of Alzheimer's disease, experts are aware of a few things. It is often viewed as a complex disease, which means many variables and behaviors might possibly contribute to its development. However, many hereditary mutations, genetic deviations that are passed through generations within families, have been determined to be one of the most prevalent and predominant genetic risk factors for the disease. Scientists describe them as autosomal dominant mutations, as they have the ability to duplicate themselves and develop deficiencies over many generations. Because of this, researchers utilize them to segregate those who possess a single copy of the mutation from those who do not. Despite the fact that sporadic versions of the disease frequently occur, such a small proportion is caused by the inheritance of genetics. Even people who do have these mutations usually acquire them from alleles of an existing condition, which represents less than 1% of all Alzheimer's diagnoses.

Alzheimer's disease is the most common form of dementia in older adults, impacting countless mental and bodily functions. It is a neurodegenerative disease that results in a loss of memory, a decreased capacity to carry out day-to-day activities, and even controlling the body. The disease is one that develops progressively, with a slow start and worsening over time. The exact cause is still unidentified, but health practitioners believe heredity, changes in the brain, and pathological changes may all be contributors.

2.1. Genetic Factors

Advances in medical genetics during the last decade and retirement of the doctrine "genes predispose, environments dispose" have shifted between them in Alzheimer's disease. When we began this chapter just a few months ago, we were struck by how little seemed to have changed axiomatically: APOE was (and apparently is) a "clinically irrelevant" pool of genetic information given fitting large enough to diagnose AD patients living in countries with high-quality healthcare. That is, whose diagnosis of AD was based agreeably as possible between and within institutions and over time. Informational practice reflects the way mainstream genetics has ignored AD and other neurodegenerative diseases, or peoples' advances since Kim's group reported the polymorphism more political predisposition to AD in 1995. These questions are complex, but it's worth laying out the genetic background to understand their surrogates.

Neuropathological findings, of course, continue to guide our understanding of Alzheimer's disease (AD). But in this chapter, we focus on genetic factors that influence thinking about the disease and its treatment. As Pathway and many other articles have made clear over the years, mutations in three genes - encoding the amyloid beta precursor protein (APP), apolipoprotein E (APOE), and an early-onset protein presenilin 1 (PSEN1) - account for a significant fraction of early- and late-onset familial AD (FAD) and sporadic AD (SAD). This is merely the first genetic fractional vapor lock that genetics has found on the road toward comprehending pathogenesis. Genetics has long been a fashion and scientific default mode to think, if not project, topoi and clichés of open-ended process, of unmapped directions, of near-infinite interactions regarding brain metabolism. But you're none of this... You are a button. A single region. A single neurotransmitter pathway. Genes.

2.2. Brain Changes and Pathology

During this time, often the brain is shrinking because the cells are generally not being replaced. When the whole brain has shrunk enough for the patient to be categorized as having advanced dementia by clinical standards, the symptoms are severe enough for families to seek professional help, by which time the nerve cell has often been irreversibly damaged and the AD processes affecting the brain's chemistry have been active for at least 20 years. Finally, the lack of activity in the brain has resulted in the brain's gradual failure to control functions such as swallowing, digesting food, maintaining our body temperature, and controlling our immune system. Brain final breakdown often takes many years and may cause increasing convulsions and loss of control of body movements, causing loss of ability to swallow, which results in death.

More than one abnormal process appears to be involved in Alzheimer's disease, which results in the death of nerve cells in the brain. Our understanding of what happens in Alzheimer's disease has changed substantially over the last decade. As a result of the failure of nerve cells to function effectively or to regenerate, patients develop increasing cognitive and functional impairments, including loss of memory, disorientation, and impaired reasoning. Later, patients may become bedridden and immobile when the damage affects the areas of the brain that control movement. Death usually occurs due to general debilitation or an intercurrent physical illness due to infections 5-20 years after the initial onset of illness. However, the underlying cause of AD is nerve cell death in the absence of injury, with the majority of the pathology in the parts of the brain responsible for our higher cognitive function. The dead neurons are replaced by protein-filled cavities called plaques.

3. Current Treatment Approaches

Pharmacological treatments only provide a degree of symptomatic relief and do not significantly modify the underlying disease process. Non-pharmacological approaches address a variety of areas including distress or discomfort, environmental modifications to reduce patient anxiety, and other aspects of daily living, such as staff training, that may improve the overall patient care situation. It is also known that addressing NPS can increase the ability to keep the patient at home for a longer period than if the NPS are unattended. A future treatment for AD may involve a combined approach that targets both the causes and symptomatic expression of the disease at the same time. While this may prove to be the best treatment approach, it may also prove to be incredibly complex both in development and practice. Current progress in research supports a more broad and individualized approach to the identification of potential new treatments. Research approaches in drug discovery include targeted preclinical biomarkers profiling, expansion in drug targets, immunotherapy, and other neurotrophic approaches.

The current treatment approaches for Alzheimer's disease (AD) are classified into two main groups: pharmacological treatments directed at the physiological or histopathological pathways affected by the AD pathology accumulating in the brain, and other treatments targeting issues related but not limited to cognition or physical health. Amongst the psychotropic drugs, antipsychotic medications are prescribed for the treatment of agitation and aggression with a high potential for injury to themselves or others, or severe self-injury. While antipsychotics are used in 27.5% of all long-term care facility residents, close to 70% of LTCF residents with AD or other dementias are on antipsychotic medications. Antipsychotics limit the patient's ability to participate or benefit from interventions designed to address the causative factors of NPS and to adjust the environment to better support the patient. Reassessing the overall health of the patient and the presence of any other medical comorbid conditions has been shown to improve the ability to taper and discontinue such medications.

3.1. Pharmacological Interventions

Likewise, the therapeutic mechanisms of memantine have been associated both with the peripheral medicinal physiological principles of ion frailty and with the inhibitory glutamatergic mechanisms that appear to possess the useful effects of reducing neuronal beta amyloid production and plaque desegregation that is seen when low levels of amyloid beta are produced or when neurofibrillary tangles are present, even when agrios are present. Donepezil, rivastigmine, galantamine, memantine, and the two used in the trials demonstrate the mechanisms after the start of cognitive deterioration seem to hold dollar with amyloid beta amyloid endocrin to same therapy and over.

Pharmacological mechanisms exploited as targets in presently available medicinal interventions to retard and ameliorate the course of AD. The currently available therapies exploit clinically significant molecular mechanisms of the CNS tissue and other internal organs. It is an established fact that there is an intimate relationship between the dysregulation of previously mentioned effector mechanisms of cholinergic and glutamatergic neurotransmissions as well as the material expression of amyloid beta and plaque neurofibrillary tangles, in both the clinical history of dementia of the Alzheimer's type, of Down people and the therapeutics of cholinesterase inhibitors.

3.2. Non-Pharmacological Interventions

Neurobiological gospel state with the adjacent neuronal formations make rapid strides, as the trade union of subspecialties in neuroscience capitalizes on talented growths. We provide cognitive lifting or physical exercises on the understanding that holistic exercise could describe experimental and clinical observations, and argue that innovative pharmacological studies in newer neuroscience findings would benefit from a similar alliance developed with leading cognitive/occupational rehabilitation or psychology researchers. It was forward-looking programs tackling the impending global pandemic that we are most likely to report on: the skyrocketing instances of Alzheimer's and dementias. Research has already shown that these programs work, so it is time to be mastering them. Moving back upstream in order to detect and treat older adults is extremely important. In this most devastating dementia type known as Alzheimer's can be presented to the right experts, perhaps new science concerning breakthrough interventions will be discovered. Sudden pushes for rigour would be more useful in psychology and bioethics. It is crucial to enhance confidentiality and to view the laws of confidentiality and nutritional research with regards to dementias. In the cyber age, laws governing childhood should be defined, in addition to cognitive screening that takes into account their tinge range. With respect to its population, AD would be seen as lethal, if mostly diabetes-mellitus-related dementias are what the neuropoverty tide turns. Critical gains for ADRD prevention will fade.

Over the past few years, several new approaches in healthcare research and treatments have been added to the therapeutic repertoire to handle Alzheimer's disease (AD). These new approaches, including some current hypotheses of AD, have already employed non-pharmacological interventions. Although not included the use of medication, these non-medical treatments constitute the subject of developing legal interest particularly concerning older people with dementia such as those with AD. This document analyses non-pharmacological treatment options in AD as thoroughly as possible for non-pharmacological interventions in all population groups. For example, this would bring a broad range of topics to the front.

4. Emerging Therapeutic Strategies

Not only has the development in the image been successful, and the crescents used in studies clear, but AD has also become a subject of focus for editors. A string of minute facts, still limited by the ethical considerations that carve the line between life and death, was publicly released. The world has been waiting for this minute informative medication with great expectance, eagerly looking forward to the achievements of the newly chosen medication. Between a hopeful utility of these emerging therapeutic strategies and the reality of being able to create a dramatic opposite in their management of the AD situation, the results of these studies will be the defining moments in the AD circumstances betrayer. One of these newly chosen medications breezes through studies and sparks the joy of researchers in order for us to be able to convince ourselves, focusing on a different class of the mix, Ti Siglu and Ti Siglu Co-Vanitac and Ti Siglu and Ten and interrelated ATB controls.

Emerging therapeutic strategies. Until fairly recently, the standard treatments for AD revolved around cholinergic drugs (initially tacrine, and subsequently donepezil, rivastigmine, and galantamine) and/or memantine. For those drugs, an effect on disease progression is questionable. Other new treatments come into sight that have a more direct effect on pathological hallmarks of AD. Immunotherapy, which stimulates or depresses the immune system, has been elaborately studied, but the clinical results so far have been disappointing. Over the last couple of years, there has been a strong build-up to examine this therapy in early phases of AD in ever-improving clinical studies. Precise medication and an approach that take individual variations in the genes of patients are therefore also heavily investigated. The coming years will without a doubt bring a range of new medications, which will improve the avenue of the fight against AD.

4.1. Immunotherapy

Recently, findings of over two dozen randomized, placebo-controlled trials reported at the Alzheimer's Association International Conference 2019 (AAIC 2019) targeting passive immunotherapies against Aβ is an accumulation of high and low molecular weight of Aβs, increase brain inflammation, enhance micro-hemorrhage and cognitive decline. Findings from the latest reports over the last year or so, however, suggest that moving to immune modulation may still be a logical step. These exciting new developments in the immunotherapy for AD show that a better understanding of the mechanisms that drive the disease is leading to the development of treatment strategies that can commandeer these mechanisms to help the body fight disease. Thirteen monoclonal antibodies (mAbs) that recognize and selectively bind to distinct conformations of Aβ epitopes have recently demonstrated inefficacy as monotherapies or immunotherapies, further confirming that targeting Aβ proteins is a failed strategy for the treatment of clinical AD.

Alzheimer's remains one of the top ten leading global causes of death, as well as the UK's leading cause of death, and yet there is no cure for AD. The current treatment strategies for AD focus on managing some of the symptoms through the use of acetylcholinesterase inhibitors or memantine for N-Methyl-D-Aspartate receptor activity. However, none of this slows disease progression or stops the disease, rendering more than 27.7 million individuals worldwide. Recent findings have totally altered our understanding of AD brain pathophysiology. Although toxic, β-amyloid will not remain as distinct toxic oligomeric forms and aggregates that are required as potential immuno-therapeutic targets. On the perpendicular front, tau pathology spreads from the entorhinal region to the entire brain transneuronally via Aβ induced tau propagation. As a result, immunotherapy is moving beyond Aβ as an immunotherapeutic target for AD patients. Consequently, the current therapeutic strategies are to delay the upstream event, i.e. tau spread throughout the brain.

4.2. Precision Medicine

This review was aimed at giving an overview of the knowledge gained on different AD phenotypes, mechanisms, and important outcomes by aggregating clinical and neuropathological data accumulated throughout a myriad of often globally oriented studies and projects, but seldom giving voice to the access patient and caregiver perspectives, frequently offering a western or high-income account of the disease. In addition, it is well illustrated that there is no longer space for a timepoint-dependent therapeutic model and that modern healthcare has to evolve to personalize its care in a structured way. So, one might say that this review retrospects, summarizing knowledge until today and heralding future advances, triggering a discussion where personalized healthcare will probably progress further to treat diseases such as Alzheimer's dementia, with which we currently struggle worldwide.

Another emerging therapeutic strategy that might well turn the current very moderate effect sizes for particular intervention targets into promising effects for a selected subgroup is precision medicine. This modern form of therapeutic interventions is built on the backbone of Glannon's 'hyper-personalized medicine'. Doing so, we first have to carefully consider those divergent forms Alzheimer's disease takes. Similarly, our knowledge of the current and etiological variables that interact, yielding particular phenotypic expressions. Hence, subgroups will be eligible for the administration of different drugs to 'cure' the disease rather than to target core symptom domains such as cognitive functioning and behavior.

5. Clinical Trials and Research Studies

Clinical trials evaluating the many promising disease modifying agents and interventions developed in the laboratory and now in the pipeline need volunteers to help determine their safety and efficacy. Clinical trials are also the research method preferred by many, who point to the Hippocratic Oath for its declaration "First, do no harm," as justifying their approach. While controversy abounds, there may not be any single best way to conduct the research. However, the individual's aspiration for quality of life serves as a universal platform for the importance of the research. It is no exaggeration that due to the size, symptoms and trajectory of the diagnosis of the disease, AD is a "get out of jail free" pass for hundreds of scientists' careers-worth of research experience. Clinical trials, research studies and preclinical and clinical pilot studies refine our understanding of AD and treatment today. Every positive, negative or anywhere-in-between result of every clinical trial or research study continues to advance our understanding of Alzheimer's disease.

For patients and families faced with an Alzheimer's disease diagnosis even as recently as 20 years ago, the notion that Alzheimer's disease is a disease with a multi-factorial etiology and potentially modifiable factors was not even part of the commonly held paradigm. Now, the number of worldwide clinical trials studying various preventions, interventions or treatments of AD is a dramatic indicator of these great changes in our understanding of AD. In the typical year over the past decade, there are between 200 and 300 actively recruiting clinical trials for AD. This dramatic increase in the number of clinical trials related to AD far outpaces the number of recruiting trials for any other neurological diagnosis.

5.1. Importance of Clinical Trials

The clinical trials report to the helmsman when sail is full, and with compass in hand, and with eye steady to the crest, the helmsman determines the next year's course. Clinical trials tell us much of the present and future, and chart a course of future study. The clinical trials in the Alzheimer field are generally done within the rubric of a given story that is already known. They are not complete surrogates for a complete understanding, nor are trials in heart disease, diabetes, cancer, and the other areas of medical research where we often complain of a lack of understanding as to the underlying cause of our infirmity. It is in the face of what we do not know that clinical trials become even more important and precious. If the present of therapeutic research in the realm of Alzheimer's disease is nicely dressed, and goes strutting mildly about, this is so largely out of the inspiration provided from others at forums such as this. And out of the laboratory. To focus on the clinical side to myopia is to invite dizziness in the amount of data that exists and also that which cannot exist because of ignorance.

Alzheimer's research is the plotted course of a sailing ship on stormy seas. From the vantage point of the present, it is easy to see the broad outline of the future and to know that, having sailed through cold, hurricane, and doldrum, a fair wind shall yet be ours. This advance to fair wind, however, is gradual and follows two Watts-perfect parallel paths. The first separates the grain of the promising seamen from the chaff of those trailed astern.

5.2. Promising Research Areas

The ex-vivo two ethics will be enacted for neurotherapeutics long prior to the emergence of any new medications through vivo tests. The ex-vivo ethics will be enabled by new brain scanning technologies as well as advances in intra-operative corticotomies (subconscious interventions)—both of which may engender the squirmy eel of nascent medical ethics in other settings—by minimally invasive neurosimulation of essential brain systems. These advances would render a range arrest with ongoing volition through formal detection of the actions of antisocial libertarians in the prefrontal cortex. Before proceeding, the primary aim is (obtaining information that would make conception of informed consent practicable, even as the defense against a response is under construction) to prevent the urgent sequestration of a military informant informed by the fiery pinkie of putative property in the air.

• Results and Ethics: Prefatory Investigations are described to construct nascent defenses for trials of brain implants using fetal tissue and stem cells. These would be controlled iterations of the procedures designed in 1987–1989 to construct two nascent medical ethics as well-regulated sin ex vivo.

• Basic Science. Neurodegenerative diseases have been difficult to tackle with new drugs. Yet the paralleling research of the past 30 years has been picking its way slowly through the neuron. So early — so base and molecular. It is hard to wait for it to accumulate into changes in care, much as it is difficult to be somewhat cancer patients cannot wait. Now, however, our wait might be beginning to turn into benefits within a few years. Nearer than stem cells, gene therapy might serve as an early holding pen for wild biological possibilities and ethical challenges. Initial trials in gene therapy, which might be hard for prisoners to refuse, might forearm the informed consent boards of the future better than stem cell trials.

Prior to "what's promising," roles and possible implications have not undergone exhaustive studies. The fact that new priorities and possibilities have been identified in relation to these forces shows the newness of these research areas. That said, our understanding of these areas lags behind, and so these explanations are preliminary and speculative. Here is a brief discussion of exemplar research areas that point toward what may be coming in the coming decade.

6. Challenges and Future Directions

Future directions will remain focused on the successful development and access to curative treatments. To achieve this, international collaborative efforts with intensive multi-disciplinary collaboration are necessary in the domains of basic biology, epidemiology, genetics, informatics, stem cell therapies, ethics, policy, clinical research, post-marketing follow up, cohort building, and clinical trial recruitment. In addition, the field calls for a paradigm shift in the neuropathology community to no longer perceive and describe other abnormal protein aggregates or co-pathologies as independent pathogenic entities. Rather, we need an integrative holistic way of evaluating the composite of neuropathologies, their staging or spreading, and recognize the relative weight of different contributor products. The lack of such composite measures serves to confuse the public and policy makers and make it difficult to carefully correlate neuropathological findings with symptoms. Differences in oxidative stress and calcium regulation between distinct neurodegenerative conditions must also be explored. The future of international initiatives in developing therapies will focus on countries and economies that have the highest burden of dementia: North America, Europe, South America, and South Asia. It is especially important that increasing numbers of people in all regions of the world enter clinical studies at very early disease states in the disease course, where brain reserve might be optimal, so that new therapies have the capability of being tested and understood for the ability to modify the disease itself.

The greatest challenge in Alzheimer's disease care and research is the tension created by the rapid advances in the development of diagnostic and therapeutic technologies and the relatively slow-paced understanding of the disease processes. This requires changes to protocols or therapeutic guidelines developed through well-designed clinical trials and many years of observation. The multi-dimensional nature of the disease offers infinite possibilities for therapeutic targets. A second ethical challenge is the collective access to level one evidence-based developed therapies and potentially curative treatments. The third ethical challenge is the access to necessary care and services. On a positive note, the field has made remarkable advances in Alzheimer's disease research and drug development over the years. Shifts in focus have led to important inroads in the understanding of the diverse risk factors for the disease.

6.1. Ethical Considerations

It is imperative that those involved in the treatment and research of individuals with AD carefully consider and prepare for the ethical and moral, as well as scientific, problems generated by the disease. Factors to consider fall into three central themes: (1) the individual with AD, (2) the individual's social milieu, and (3) global implications. AD touches every ethical and social practice and area. While these areas will always be interconnected, it strengthens the focus of the general commentary to categorize them in this manner.

Young-onset AD poses moral dilemmas for health professionals, institutions, and policymakers. The disease is less common but more aggressive in its onset, and many cases are linked to autosomal dominant familial mutations. It emerges at a time when family units are frequently breaking apart, and when responsibilities for raising children still reside predominantly with young parents. Furthermore, young adults are generally healthier and have more trusting attitudes towards other human beings and social institutions. Even middle-aged people often struggle to garner the maturational wisdom of aging; they are generally more impulsive and aggressive and have, on average, significantly more complex social and economic commitment matrices. Consequently, AD beginning before the age of 65 can have particularly severe community, individual, and family-devastating effects.

Ethics

6.2. Access to Care and Resources

Many groups, including women, those who are generally from racial/ethnic minority populations, and/or have low education attainment, are less likely to be diagnosed with AD. That means that people who may need early intervention or treatments have a longer duration with undiagnosed AD which may ultimately affect the effectiveness of available treatments. Furthermore, there are pockets of systemic racism, ethnocentrism, and plant at multiple levels of healthcare delivery that contribute to boroughs in disease diagnosis, treatments, and death, including higher rates of ADs. A 2022 report on the global prevention and treatment of AD emphasizes the need to address access to general medical, psychiatric, and mental health care and access to comprehensive long-term supports and services. It urges increased funding for promoting health behaviors that may delay or prevent the onset of AD and emphasizes reducing disparities in access to care and resources as fundamental to reducing the impact of AD.

The consequences of AD are not only experienced by the individual with the disease, but also by the caregivers, loved ones, and healthcare providers. Because many individuals with AD require long-term care from caregivers either at home or in residential facilities, individuals around the world need access to care and resources. It is estimated that 53% worldwide and 65% in Europe of people with dementia lack a diagnosis. In addition, it has been estimated that only 10-30% of individuals in low- to middle-income countries and 50% or fewer of individuals in high-income countries are diagnosed with dementia. Even within high-income countries, such as the United States, access to timely diagnoses and personalized treatment and care are not universal irrespective of payer sources.

7. Conclusion

Scientists and clinicians are putting together a more enriched comprehension of how Alzheimer's disease starts and advances. In the end, these prevalence numbers will possibly increase significantly, and new biomarkers, along with more recent pharmaceutical ideas, will hopefully bring early diagnosis and prevention services to people at risk. In addition, in a limited group of individuals, studies with new medications are underway based on these newly identified variables. Acute concomitant illnesses in the elderly, such as infection with COVID-19, result in increased dangerous exacerbations of cognitive problems and death; these episodes can cause long-term morbidity in previously resilient Alzheimer's brains. Several teams are using artificial intelligence and a combination of certain genetic traits and environmental variables to assess a new interdependence risk component. The ubiquitous gene-based pillar of developing AD is a portion of this fresh research paradigm, with a suggested therapeutic strategy that has evolved focusing on common polygenic factors, the mechanisms behind the resilience of some folks that results from constructive transactional activity across the entire average lifetime. Monitoring and predicting cognitive declines in asymptomatic elderly—and providing medications to preemptively prevent or slow their progression—will become more and more tense scenarios. Whether it's with amyloid-improved PET scans or other markers, as well as anti-amyloid, anti-tau, or anti-inflammatory medications in various phases, this strategy is multiplying into thousands of people across the globe who are involved in careful testing. Resilience must eventually integrate various potentials and genetic traits—age, gender, and obviously cultural and ethnic origins. Management, care and quality of life, and resilience of the population suffering from AD depend profoundly on this understanding. In this complicated field of collateral research aspects, the final authorizing layer ultimately rests with bioethics, law, psychology, and social sciences in general.